The Complete Women's Guide to Preventing Breast Cancer

Dani Raymond

Table of Content

<u>Chapter 7: Additional Information Sources</u>

<u>Conclusion</u>

Introduction

A. The Importance of Breast Health: Nurturing Wellness and Preventing Breast Cancer

For women's entire quality of life and general well-being, breast health is a crucial concern. Intricate structures that need adequate care and attention, a woman's breasts are more than just a representation of femininity. Reducing the risk of breast cancer and ensuring early detection are as important as embracing self-care in terms of understanding the significance of breast health.

We will examine all of the important factors of breast health, including anatomy, precautions, and the value of early detection.

Breast Anatomy: The Basis of Well-being

Understanding the female breast's anatomy is crucial to appreciating the significance of breast health. Fatty, connective, and glandular tissue make up the breasts. The glandular tissue consists of ducts that carry milk to the nipple and lobules that produce milk. While fatty tissue gives the breast more volume, connective tissue supports the structure.

Knowing the anatomy of the breasts enables women to be in tune with their bodies and track any changes. Breast health requires regular self-breast inspections as well as knowledge of typical breast changes during the menstrual cycle. These procedures aid in locating any odd lumps, skin alterations, or discharge from the nipples that might indicate a problem.

Breast Health and Risk Reduction

Since several factors might raise one's risk of developing breast cancer, breast health and risk reduction go hand in hand. Finding and changing these risk factors is essential for prevention. Better lifestyle choices can help to enhance breast health, but genetics and other risk factors are unavoidable.

1. Diet and Nutrition: Rich in fruits, vegetables, and lean proteins, a well-balanced diet helps promote breast health. These foods' antioxidants and phytochemicals may help shield cells from harm and lower the risk of cancer.

2. Physical Activity: Exercise regularly is associated with a lower risk of breast cancer. In addition to aiding with weight management, exercise may also have an impact on hormone levels, which may raise the risk of breast cancer.

3. Stress and Sleep: Prolonged stress and inadequate sleep have a

detrimental effect on general health, which includes breast health. A healthy lifestyle must include both stress reduction strategies and enough sleep.

4. Alcohol and Smoking: Reducing alcohol intake and quitting smoking are important strategies for lowering the risk of breast cancer. There is evidence linking smoking and alcohol use to a higher risk of breast cancer.

Early Detection

It is crucial to recognize problems with breast health early on and to take action. Treatment results and survival rates are considerably improved by early identification of breast cancer.

Mammogram clinical breast exams: are self-breast inspection routines or ways that women can take control of their breast health.

Self-Breast Exams: Self-breast exams are a straightforward but useful method for early detection. Women can do these examinations at home by feeling their breast tissue for any lumps or changes. Self-examination regularly provides the chance to identify problems early on.

Clinical Breast Exams: A medical professional's clinical breast exam offers a more comprehensive evaluation of breast health. Women of all ages are advised to do it since medical professionals are qualified to identify minute alterations that self-examinations can miss.

Mammograms: Mammography is a type of specialized breast X-ray that can identify cancers that are too tiny to feel. Frequent mammograms are essential for early detection and prevention, particularly for women over 40.

Risk Factor and Genetic Testing

Even while there are risk factors that are beyond of control, being aware of one's personal risk profile can be powerful. To determine their vulnerability, women with a family history of breast cancer can think about undergoing genetic testing.

Genetic testing can detect BRCA1 and BRCA2 gene mutations that raise the risk of breast cancer. With this information at hand, people are more equipped to make decisions regarding their health, such as stepping up surveillance and taking preventative action.

Support and Education

Breast health includes only physical health but also psychological and emotional support. Women who receive a breast cancer diagnosis need a solid support network because the news can be emotionally taxing. People can get support through support groups, counseling, and instructional materials while they negotiate the challenging process of receiving a breast cancer diagnosis and treatment.

In conclusion, a crucial component of women's general well-being is breast health. It's important to know the anatomy of the breasts, make educated lifestyle decisions, and keep an eye on your breast health. By detecting breast cancer in its earliest, most treatable stages, early diagnosis through self-breast checks, clinical exams, and mammography can save lives.

Furthermore, being aware of risk factors and genetic testing enables people to make well-informed decisions regarding their health. Women who prioritize their breast health can cultivate wellness, lower their risk of breast cancer, and ultimately lead longer happier lives. Breast health is a lifelong endeavor.

B. Breast Cancer Overview: Understanding a Common Health Concern

Breast cancer is a common and serious health issue that primarily affects women, however, it can also strike men. A thorough understanding of breast cancer is essential to addressing this problem and promoting breast health. We'll go over the fundamentals of breast cancer in this summary, including its definition, kinds, risk factors, and the significance of early identification.

Defining Breast Cancer

Cancer that starts in the breast's cells is known as breast cancer. It happens when a malignant tumor forms as a result of a disruption in the regular, regulated process of cell growth and division. The term "metastasis" refers to the ability of these malignant cells to infiltrate surrounding tissues and possibly spread to other areas of the body.

Types of Breast Cancer

Breast cancer is a collection of many cancer forms that attack the breast rather than a single illness. The following are the most typical forms of breast cancer:

1. Ductal Carcinoma In Situ (DCIS): DCIS is a type of non-invasive breast cancer in which aberrant cells are discovered in the duct lining but have not yet moved to the outside of it.

2. Breast cancer of the invasive ductal carcinoma (IDC) variety is the most prevalent kind. It begins in a milk duct, penetrates the wall of the duct, and spreads across the surrounding breast tissue.

3. Invasive Lobular Carcinoma (ILC): ILC can spread to surrounding tissues

after starting in the breast's milk-producing lobules.

4. Triple-negative breast cancer: Treatment for this type of cancer is more difficult since it lacks three specific receptors (progesterone, estrogen, and HER2).

5. HER2-Positive Breast Cancer: Cells with this type of cancer overexpress HER2, a protein that can stimulate the proliferation of cancer cells.

6. Inflammatory Breast Cancer: This is a rare but assertive type of breast cancer characterized by redness and swelling of the breast.

Breast Cancer Risk Factors

Several risk factors can raise the possibility of breast cancer. It's important to understand these factors for prevention and early detection:

1. Gender: While breast cancer can strike anybody, women are far more likely to have it than males.

2. Age: Women over 50 are more likely than any other age group to have breast cancer.

3. Family History: Having a close relative with a history of breast cancer can increase the risk.

4. Genetic Mutations: Genes such as BRCA1 and BRCA2 that have inherited

mutations can greatly raise the risk of breast cancer.

5. Hormone Replacement Therapy (HRT): There may be an increased risk associated with some kinds of HRT, especially a combination of estrogen and progesterone therapy.

6. Radiation Exposure: There may be a higher risk if there has been prior chest radiation exposure, particularly in childhood or adolescence.

7. Lifestyle Factors: Adopting unhealthy habits like smoking and binge drinking can raise your chance of developing breast cancer.

The Importance of Early Detection

When it comes to effective treatment and survival, early detection of breast cancer is crucial. Mammograms, clinical breast exams, and self-breast inspections are essential for detecting breast cancer in its early, most curable stages.

Self-breast exams enable people to keep an eye on the health of their breasts and notify medical specialists right away if there are any changes or anomalies. Healthcare professionals' clinical breast exams provide a more thorough assessment. Mammography, a type of specialist X-ray imaging of the breast, is capable of identifying cancers that are too small to feel during a physical examination.

In summary, breast cancer is a complicated and common health issue that primarily affects women. It impacts a large number of people. In the fight against this disease, knowledge of the various forms, risk factors, and the significance of early detection is crucial. We can improve the lives of people impacted by breast cancer by making progress in prevention, early identification, and effective treatment via ongoing research, education, and proactive measures.

C. The Aim of this Book: The Complete Women's Guide to Preventing Breast Cancer

This book aims to provide women with the information and techniques necessary to take charge of their breast health and lower their chance of developing breast cancer. The goal of this book is to serve as a thorough guide for women seeking to improve their breast health by providing information, inspiration, and support.

1. Education and Awareness: The goal of the book is to inform women about the significance of breast health, including the anatomy of the breasts, risk factors, and forms of breast cancer. It gives users the basic information they need to make knowledgeable decisions about their health by presenting information understandably and straightforwardly.

2. Prevention and Risk Reduction: Helping women make lifestyle decisions that lower their chance of developing breast cancer is one of the book's main goals. This covers talks about physical activity, stress reduction, nutrition and diet, and other preventive measures. The book gives readers the tools they need to take proactive actions to safeguard their breast health by providing useful guidance and doable steps.

3. Early Screening and Detection: The book emphasizes how important early detection is to enhancing the prognosis of breast cancer patients. To help women monitor their breast health and seek early screening when needed, it offers comprehensive information on clinical breast exams,

self-breast examinations, and mammography. Through highlighting the need for early detection, the book hopes to improve outcomes and increase survival rates.

4. Resources and Support: Coping with breast cancer can be an emotionally and physically taxing experience. The purpose of this book is to provide information and assistance to women who are coping with breast cancer or who wish to assist a loved one. It contains survivor testimonies and experiences, support group information, and links to resources for more training and help.

5. Empowerment: The main goal of the book is to give women more authority. It empowers people to take charge of

their health, make wise choices, and have faith in their capacity to safeguard and preserve their breast health. The book helps women become champions for their well-being by arming them with information and practical tactics.

In conclusion, "The Complete Women's Guide to Preventing Breast Cancer " is an invaluable resource that empowers women to take control of their breast health rather than only being a book. The mission is to empower, educate, and assist women on their path to a future free of cancer.

The goal of this book is to improve women's lives by preventing and early identifying breast cancer through the

dissemination of critical knowledge
and techniques.

Chapter 1: Understanding Breast Cancer

A . Fundamentals of Breast Anatomy: Understanding the Basis for Breast Health

Understanding the fundamentals of breast anatomy is crucial to appreciating the significance of breast health. The female breast is a multipurpose, intricate tissue that produces milk and provides nourishment for her babies. The basis for identifying any alterations or anomalies and preserving general breast health is an understanding of breast anatomy. We'll look at the essential elements of breast anatomy here.

Breast Structure

Three main types of tissue make up the breast:

1. Glandular Tissue: Known as the breast's functional tissue, is what produces milk. It consists of lobules, which are collections of microscopic sacs that make milk, and a system of ducts that carry the milk to the nipple.

2. Tissue Connective: Tissue connective tissue gives the breasts structural stability. It consists of fibrous tissue and ligaments that

support the preservation of the position and form of the breast.

3. Adipose tissue, sometimes referred to as fatty tissue, envelops the connective and glandular tissues. It fluctuates in quantity and gives the breast more volume.

Dumps and Lobules

The little milk-producing organs in the breast called lobules resemble grapes. These lobules activate during pregnancy and lactation and produce milk. Next, the milk travels via a system of ducts, which resemble tiny tubes. The nipple, the site of lactation release during nursing, is where these ducts converge.

Lymphatic and Blood Vessels

The breast is full of blood arteries that feed the glandular tissue with nutrition and oxygen. The breast also contains lymphatic vessels, which are essential to the immune system of the body. The lymphatic system aids in the removal of waste materials and extra fluid from breast tissue.

Nipple and Areola

Encircling the nipple, in a circular pattern, is the areola. The elevated, central area of the breast where milk is released during nursing is called the nipple. The stimulation of milk release and sexual arousal is largely dependent on the many nerve endings found in the areola and nipple.

Breasts change throughout Life

A Woman's breast architecture changes during her life, mostly due to variations in hormone levels. Breast tissue grows and matures during puberty. Hormonal fluctuations during the menstrual cycle can result in transient breast changes including soreness or edema.

The glandular tissue of the breast undergoes major alterations throughout pregnancy as it gets ready to produce milk. The composition of breast tissue changes after menopause, with an increase in fatty tissue and a decrease in glandular tissue.

It is essential to comprehend these typical alterations to identify any anomalous developments. Women can discern between potential health risks related to their breasts and typical hormonal swings by regularly self-examining their breasts and being aware of these differences.

In conclusion, glandular, connective, and fatty tissue make up the intricate and multipurpose structure that is the female breast. The breast produces milk and provides immunity through a network of ducts, blood arteries, and lymphatic vessels. Understanding these basic features of breast anatomy is necessary to keep an eye on breast health and spot any abnormalities, which is important for the early detection and prevention of breast cancer and other breast-related problems.

B. What is breast cancer?

Understanding the Complexities of a Common Disease: Breast Cancer

Cancer that starts in the breast's cells is known as breast cancer. The unchecked proliferation and division of aberrant cells within the breast tissue is its defining feature. A tumor is defined as a bulge or lump that develops from these malignant cells. Studying breast cancer entails learning about all of its facets, such as its forms, stages, causes, and the significance of early identification.

Causes of Breast Cancer

The specific cause of breast cancer is not always known, several established risk factors cause a person's chance of getting the disease. Among these risk factors are:

1. Gender: While breast cancer can strike anybody, women are significantly more likely to have it than males. Hormonal variables and the existence of breast tissue are to blame for this.

2. Age: Women over 50 are most likely to develop breast cancer, and the risk rises with age.

3. Family History: If there are known genetic alterations, a family history of breast cancer, especially in close relatives, can increase the risk.

4. Genetic Mutations: Certain genetic mutations, such as those in the BRCA1 and BRCA2 genes, considerably raise the risk of breast cancer in some people.

5. Hormone Replacement Therapy: There has been a link between a higher risk and some forms of HRT, especially the combination of estrogen and progesterone therapy.

6. Radiation Exposure: There may be a higher risk if there has been prior chest radiation exposure, particularly in childhood or adolescence.

6. Lifestyle Factors: Adopting unhealthy habits like smoking and binge drinking can raise your chance of developing breast cancer.

Types of Breast Cancer

Breast cancer is a multifactorial illness with many subtypes, each with unique features. Common kinds consist of:

1. Ductal Carcinoma In Situ (DCIS): A non-invasive cancer where abnormal cells are restricted to the lining of a breast duct.

2. Invasive Ductal Carcinoma (IDC): The most typical type, characterized by cancer cells cracking through the duct wall and invading nearby tissues.

3. Invasive Lobular Carcinoma (ILC): Originating in the milk-producing lobules, it can circulate to adjacent tissues.

4. Triple-negative breast cancer: This variety can be more difficult to treat since it lacks three specific receptors (progesterone, estrogen, and HER2).

5. HER2-Positive Breast Cancer: This type of cancer is characterized by an overabundance of the protein HER2, which stimulates the proliferation of cancer cells.

6. Breast swelling and redness are hallmarks of the uncommon but aggressive kind of breast cancer known as inflammatory breast cancer.

C. Breast Cancer Stages

The stage of breast cancer is determined by how far along it has progressed. The staging process aids in directing treatment choices. There are four stages in the cancer spectrum: o is non-invasive, and IV is an advanced stage where the disease has spread to other organs.

The Importance of Early Detection

A successful course of therapy and higher survival rates for breast cancer patients depend heavily on early detection. Mammograms, clinical breast exams, and routine self-breast exams are important diagnostic tools for detecting breast cancer in its early, most curable stages.

Breast cancer is a complicated illness with a range of risk factors, forms, and stages. Although it can affect anyone, being aware of these factors is essential to early discovery and successful treatment. Informed and proactive approaches to breast health can help people lower their risk and increase the likelihood of a favorable result in the event of a breast cancer diagnosis.

D. Statistics and risk factors

Statistics on Breast Cancer Risk: Recognizing Vulnerabilities and Prevalence

A serious health issue that mostly affects women and, to a lesser extent, males is breast cancer. Understanding the risk factors and data related to this illness is crucial to making well-informed decisions on early detection and prevention.

Statistics for Breast Cancer

Decision-making and public health awareness depend on having a thorough understanding of the incidence and consequences of breast cancer. The following are some significant breast cancer statistics:

1. Breast cancer is the most prevalent type of cancer in women worldwide. With hundreds of thousands of new cases each year, it is the most commonly diagnosed cancer in the United States.

2. Death: Although the incidence is significant, breakthroughs in treatment and early identification have led to a steady decline in the death rate. A growing number of women with breast cancer are becoming long-term survivors, and survival rates are rising.

3. Age and Risk: As people age, they are more susceptible to breast cancer. Women 50 years of age and older account for the majority of instances.

4. Genetic Elements: Hereditary factors, such as BRCA1 and BRCA2 genetic mutations, account for 5–10% of occurrences of breast cancer.

5. Screening and Early Detection: An important component of early detection is routine mammography screening. The 5-year survival rate is nearly 100% in cases of early detection, localized breast cancer detection.

6. Breast cancer has an impact on people worldwide. It is a worldwide health issue, so it is imperative to

make screening and treatment more accessible as well as to increase public awareness.

7. Survival: A large number of women who receive a breast cancer diagnosis go on to lead long, healthy lives. Quality of life and survival have grown in importance in the treatment of breast cancer.

In conclusion, breast cancer is a common, complicated illness with a wide range of risk factors and important ramifications for public health. People can lower their risk and be cautious about early identification by being aware of these risk factors and keeping up to date on breast cancer statistics. This will increase their chances of receiving a successful treatment and long-term survival.

Chapter 2: Early Detection Saves Lives

A . The Importance of Early Breast Cancer Detection:

Reducing the disease's physical and psychological effects, raising survival rates, and enhancing treatment outcomes all depend on early detection of breast cancer. Promoting breast health and lessening the effects of breast cancer requires an understanding of the importance of early detection. Here are some major justifications for the significance of early detection:

1. Higher Rates of Survival:

- The 5-year survival rate is nearly 100% in cases of early, localized breast cancer detection (Stage 0 or Stage I). Accordingly, most women with early-stage breast cancer could anticipate living a cancer-free life for a minimum of five years following their diagnosis.

2. Smaller Cancers and Simpler Therapy:

-The discovery of tiny tumors is frequently the result of early detection. Smaller tumors usually require less severe therapies or major procedures, which lessens the patient's physical and psychological load.

3. Reduced Spread:

- Early detection reduces the likelihood that breast cancer will have spread to adjacent lymph nodes or distant organs. As a result, less severe therapies including radiation and chemotherapy are required.

4. Additional Therapy Choices:

A greater range of therapeutic options, such as lumpectomy surgery, which preserves breast tissue instead of removing it entirely, are available for early-stage breast cancer. Possessing additional options for therapy improves the likelihood of retaining breast tissue as well as a woman's sense of self and body image.

5. Decreased Chance of Recurrence:

- Appropriate diagnosis and treatment lower the risk of cancer recurrence. It lessens the likelihood that cancer cells left over from the initial therapy would reappear later.

6. Life Quality:

-Early detection of breast cancer can help patients have a higher quality of life. Less aggressive treatments frequently result in fewer side effects and a quicker recovery.

7. Psychological and Emotional Health:

-Early detection of cancer helps reduce stress and anxiety related to the diagnosis. A patient's mental health may benefit from knowing that their cancer is still in its early stages and may even be cured.

8. Economy of Scale:

- Early detection may be more economical for patients and medical systems alike. Compared to advanced-stage instances that need rigorous therapy, treating early-stage breast cancer is frequently less expensive.

9. Less Forceful Interventions:

- More aggressive treatments, which might have serious side effects, can be necessary for advanced-stage breast cancer. Early identification makes it possible to employ less intrusive therapies with tolerable side effects.

10. Enhanced Knowledge and Protest:

- Campaigns and initiatives for early detection have increased public awareness of breast health. Early detection fosters a proactive health management culture by supporting routine breast self-examinations, clinical breast exams, and mammograms.

It is impossible to overestimate the importance of early breast cancer identification. It not only saves lives but also lessens the financial, emotional, and physical toll that the illness takes. People can safeguard their breast health and well-being by being proactive and actively engaged in screening and self-examination procedures. This involves knowing the significance of early detection.

B. Self-breast assessment manual

Self-Breast Examination Manual: A Comprehensive Guide to Tracking Your Breast Health

A vital component of early breast cancer detection is routine self-breast exams. You can get to know your breast tissue, spot any changes, and quickly notify your healthcare physician by doing a self-examination at home. The following is a detailed how-to guide for performing a self-breast examination:

Step 1: Get ready

- Look for a peaceful, well-lit space where you may easily stand or sit in front of a mirror.

- Take off your clothes starting at the waist and cover one breast with a towel or piece of cloth.

Step Two: Visual Inspection

1. Position Yourself Before the Mirror:

- With your arms by your sides, examine your breasts in the mirror. Examine your breasts from various perspectives, keeping an eye out for any variations in their symmetry, size, or form.

- Take note of any puckering, dimpling, or textural changes in the skin.

2. Lift Your Arms:

Raise your arms above your head and look again for any changes you see in your breasts.

3. Analyze Every Nipple:

- Examine your nipples for indications of redness, inversion (pushing inward), or discharge.

Step 3: Inspection by Hand

4. Laying Flat:

- Place a folded towel or cushion under your right shoulder while lying on your back.

- Examine your left breast with your right hand. Using your middle three fingers, push your hand flat against your breast with light, even pressure.

- Work your fingers in a clockwise circle around your breast, starting from the outside and moving progressively in the direction of the nipple.

- Continue in this manner, varying the pressure to feel the breast tissue at different depths.

-Observe any lumps, thickening, or strange textures.

5. Swap Out Position:

- Place your left hand over your right breast and repeat the check while shifting the pillow or towel to your left shoulder.

Step Four: Standing or Sitting

6. Examine While Sitting or Standing:

- Keep your arms by your sides while you stand or sit upright.

- Raise your right arm and examine your right breast with your left hand in the same circular motion as before.

6. Swap Out Position:

- Using your right hand, repeat the procedure for your left breast.

Step 5: Examining the areola and breasts

8. Examining the areola and breasts: Squeeze each nipple gently to feel for any discharge, and look for any changes in texture or color.

Examine the black region surrounding the nipple, known as the areola, for any odd lumps or changes.

Step 6: Last Actions

9. Recur Every Month:

- Once a month, or even a few days after your monthly cycle when your breasts are less likely to be sore or swollen, do this self-breast check.

10. Keep Note of Any Findings:

Record your monthly self-examinations in a journal, noting any deviations or changes.
See your doctor for a clinical breast exam or further testing if you observe any persistent changes.

Keep in mind that self-breast inspections do not serve as a replacement for routine mammograms and clinical breast exams. Combining these complementary techniques increases the likelihood of early identification and effective treatment of breast cancer.

If you see any strange changes during your self-examination, don't hesitate to consult a healthcare professional as early detection is vital. You can significantly improve your well-being by taking a proactive approach to breast health.

C. The function of mammography

Mammography's Place in Breast Health: An Essential Instrument for Early Detection

One essential diagnostic method for breast health is mammography. It is a crucial part of breast cancer screening and diagnosis, and it plays a major role in early detection of the disease. Here is a summary of the important function that mammograms play in breast health:

1. Early Identification of Disturbances:

- Mammograms are a very useful tool for identifying abnormalities of the breast, such as tumors, cysts, and other tissue alterations.

- Abnormalities that are too tiny to feel during a clinical breast exam or self-breast inspection can frequently be found by mammography.

2. Women's Asymptomatic Screening:

Mammography is a useful diagnostic technique for early detection of breast cancer because it is the primary use for these images.

- Women should have screening mammograms regularly, preferably beginning at age 40. However, depending on personal risk factors and medical advice, recommendations may change.

3. Instrument for Diagnosing Patients with Symptoms:

A woman or her healthcare practitioner may use mammography as a diagnostic technique if she notices changes in her breasts or symptoms such as pain, discharge from the nipples, or lumps.

- Diagnostic mammography offers a more thorough evaluation to identify the underlying cause of these symptoms.

4. Two types of Mammograms

- Screening and diagnostic mammography are the two main categories of mammograms.

To identify cancer early on, screening mammography is a standard exam for women who do not exhibit any symptoms.

- When there are any concerns, such as a lump or other breast abnormalities, diagnostic mammography is more thorough and performed. They offer a close-up image of a particular breast region.

5. Digital Breast Imaging:

Digital mammography has been the norm in recent years. It makes it possible to capture photos more quickly, store them more easily, and edit and modify them for better interpretation.

- High-resolution images from digital mammography can be very helpful in spotting minute anomalies.

6. 3D Tomosynthesis Mammography:

- 3D mammography, also known as tomosynthesis, is a sophisticated imaging method that builds a 3D reconstruction of the breast by taking several pictures from various perspectives.

- By producing sharper and more detailed images, this technology can improve early cancer detection and lower the likelihood of false positives.

7.   Mammography   and   Prompt Identification:

-Mammography-based early detection of breast cancer greatly enhances treatment results and survival rates.

-Early   detection   and   targeted treatment can effectively treat cancer when detected in its early, confined stages.

- Mammography offers the chance for preventive interventions because it can identify changes like calcifications, which may suggest precancerous diseases.

8. In addition to clinical examinations:

- Self-breast exams and clinical breast exams benefit greatly from the addition of mammography. Together, these methods form an all-encompassing strategy for breast health.

9. Monitoring and Follow-Up:

-Mammograms can be useful in the post-treatment follow-up of patients with breast cancer. They support the tracking of any new anomalies or recurrences.

Mammograms are essential resources for breast health. They play a crucial role in the timely identification of breast cancer and offer vital data for both screening and diagnosis. Frequent mammograms provide a holistic approach to breast health that enables people to safeguard their health and identify breast cancer at its most treatable stage, in conjunction with clinical breast exams and self-breast checks.

Chapter 3: Healthy Lifestyle Decisions

A. Nutrition and diet for healthy breasts

Nutrition and Diet for Breast Health: Boosting Your Immune System

The foundation of proper nutrition and a balanced diet is breast health. Although food alone cannot completely prevent breast cancer, it can greatly lower the risk and improve general health.

The following is a guide to the food selections and nutritional guidelines that support breast health:

1. Produce and Fruits:

- Eat a range of vibrant fruits and vegetables, including tomatoes, leafy greens, citrus fruits, berries, and carrots.

- The abundance of antioxidants, vitamins, and minerals in these foods helps shield cells from harm and lowers the chance of cancer.

2. Fiber:

- Include foods high in fiber in your diet, such as vegetables, whole grains, beans, and lentils.

- Fiber lowers the risk of breast cancer by supporting digestive function and helping with weight management.

3. Tight Protein:

- Opt for lean protein sources such as fish, chicken, beans, and legumes.

-Reducing your intake of red meat, especially grilled and processed meats may raise your chance of developing breast cancer.

4. Nutritious Fats:

- Choose healthy fats, such as those in avocados, nuts, seeds, and olive oil.

- Reduce your intake of processed and fried foods that include saturated and trans fats, as these foods may raise your risk of breast cancer.

5. The Fatty Acids Omega-3:

- Incorporate omega-3 fatty acid sources such as walnuts, flaxseeds, and fatty fish (salmon, mackerel).

- The anti-inflammatory qualities of omega-3s may lower the incidence of breast cancer.

6. Limit your intake of sugar and refined carbs.

-Cut back on the amount of sugar-filled drinks, candies, and meals prepared with white flour.

-Increased consumption of refined carbs and sugars may exacerbate inflammation and weight gain, two conditions that increase the risk of breast cancer.

7. Natural estrogens:

- Foods high in phytoestrogens, such as soy-based products, may offer some protection against breast cancer.

However, if you're worried about the link between soy consumption and the risk of breast cancer, speak with a doctor.

8. Vitamin D and calcium:

- Make sure you're getting enough calcium and vitamin D, as these nutrients help to keep your breast tissue healthy.

-Green leafy vegetables, dairy products, and fortified plant-based milk are excellent sources of calcium; supplements and sunshine are good sources of vitamin D.

9. Rich in Antioxidants Foods:

-Antioxidants found in berries, almonds, and green tea help shield cells from harm.

- Antioxidants may lower the risk of cancer and improve general health.

10. Limit alcoholic beverages:

- If you consume alcohol, do it sparingly. Since drinking alcohol has been associated with a higher risk of breast cancer, it is best to minimize or stay away from it.

11. hydration

- Drink plenty of water, herbal teas, and sugar-free drinks to stay hydrated. Sufficient hydration promotes general health.

12. Control of Portion:

- Since being overweight is a known risk factor for breast cancer, pay attention to portion sizes to help control calorie intake and maintain a healthy weight.

13. Hold on to a Healthy Weight:

- Use a balanced diet and frequent exercise to help you reach and stay at a healthy weight.

14. Aspects of Lifestyle:

- Incorporate an active lifestyle with a healthy diet, as frequent exercise can further lower the risk of breast cancer.

15. Speak with a Healthcare Professional:

-See a registered dietitian or other healthcare professional for individualized advice if you have any specific dietary issues or inquiries regarding breast health.

In conclusion, maintaining adequate nutrition and a balanced diet are essential for maintaining breast health and lowering the risk of breast cancer. People can empower their bodies to better protect against breast cancer and boost general well-being by eating well-informed foods and leading healthy lives.

B. Benefits of Exercise

Exercise's Beneficial Effects on Breast Health: Improving Well-Being and Lowering Risk

Exercise and physical activity regularly provide numerous advantages for general health, and they have a particularly favorable effect on breast health. Here's a summary of how physical activity can improve health and lower the risk of breast cancer:

1. Maintaining Weight:
- Consistent exercise contributes to a healthy body weight. Having too much body fat increases the risk of breast cancer, particularly after menopause.

- By generating calories and increasing lean muscle mass, exercise aids in weight management.

2. Hormone Control:

- Exercise helps control hormones, such as estrogen, which is linked to the onset of breast cancer.

-Regular exercise can potentially lessen the risk of breast cancer by lowering the body's estrogen levels.

3. Immune System Assistance:

- Physical activity strengthens the immune system, improving its capacity to fend against cancerous cells.

- A robust immune system lowers the likelihood of developing cancer by being better able to recognize and eradicate aberrant cells.

4. Cut Down on Inflammation:

- Several illnesses, including cancer, are associated with chronic inflammation.

-Engaging in regular exercise can aid in the reduction of chronic inflammation, potentially lowering the risk of breast cancer.

5. Sensitivity to Insulin:

- Exercise raises insulin sensitivity and lowers the risk of type 2 diabetes and insulin resistance.

- Exercise plays a crucial role in the prevention of diabetes since high insulin levels are linked to a higher risk of breast cancer.

6. Improved Airflow:

- Improved blood circulation brought about by exercise guarantees that nutrients and oxygen reach the breast tissues effectively.

-Enhanced circulation can lessen oxidative stress and promote tissue repair, both of which are important for breast health.

7. A decrease in breast density

- Frequent exercise can reduce breast density, which can improve the ability of mammograms to identify breast abnormalities.

8. Mental Health and Wellness:

- Physical activity improves mental health by lowering stress, anxiety, and depressive symptoms.

- Emotional stability and a positive outlook can support general health and wellness.

9. Function of Lymphatic System:

- Exercise promotes the lymphatic system's smooth operation, which facilitates the elimination of waste materials and poisons from breast tissues.

- This is necessary to keep your breasts functioning normally.

10. Bone Wellness:

- Activities that require bearing weight, including strength training and walking, are good for the health of your bones.

- Keeping your bones strong is important for your general health and can lower your chance of fractures and some diseases, such as breast cancer.

11. Support therapy:

- Exercise can be included in a comprehensive treatment plan for people who have already been diagnosed with breast cancer.

- It can enhance the quality of life, lessen the chance of cancer recurrence, and assist in managing the negative effects of cancer treatments.

12. Prevention of Breast Cancer:

-Research indicates that women who participate in consistent, moderate-to-intense physical exercise are at a lower risk of breast cancer.

- To prevent breast cancer, the American Cancer Society suggests engaging in at least 150 minutes of moderate-intensity exercise or 75 minutes of vigorous-intensity exercise every week.

13. Tailored to Meet Specific Needs:

It is possible to customize exercise to a person's preferences and level of fitness. Everyone can find something they enjoy doing, whether it's weight training, yoga, swimming, or strolling.

In conclusion, there is a significant effect that exercise has on breast health. Frequent exercise improves general health and lowers the chance of breast cancer dramatically. People can empower themselves to improve their overall well-being and breast health by keeping a balanced, healthy lifestyle and adding exercise to their daily routines.

C. Managing stress and sleep

Managing Stress and Sleep for Optimal Breast Health

Effective stress management and excellent sleep are crucial components of overall well-being and play a vital role in preserving breast health. Here's why they are important and ways for controlling stress and enhancing sleep:

Stress Management:

1. Impact on Breast Health:

- Chronic stress can lead to hormonal imbalances, including elevated levels of cortisol, which may contribute to breast cancer risk.

- Stress can weaken the immune system, making the body less effective at identifying and eliminating aberrant cells.

2. Strategies for Managing Stress:

- Regular Exercise: Physical activity is a significant stress reliever. It helps release endorphins, which are natural mood lifters.

- Mindfulness and Relaxation Techniques: Practices like meditation, deep breathing, and gradual muscle relaxation can help alleviate stress.

- Time management: Having a good time management strategy might help you feel less stressed out by your daily to-do list.

- Social Support: Establishing and preserving a solid network of friends and family members can help offer emotional support during trying times.

- Counseling or therapy: Talking with a therapist can teach people constructive coping mechanisms for stressful situations.

3. Restful Sleep:

1. Impact on Breast Health:

- Several medical disorders, including breast cancer, are linked to inadequate sleep.

- The body needs sleep to repair and replace cells, including breast tissue cells.

4. Methods for Increasing Sleep Quality:

- Maintain a Regular Sleep Schedule: Even on the weekends, go to bed and wake up at the same time every day.

- Establish a relaxing Bedtime Routine: Before going to sleep, engage in relaxing activities like reading, having a warm bath, or practicing relaxation methods.

- Limit Screen Time: To prevent blue light from disrupting your sleep, avoid using displays (such as phones, computers, and TVs) just before bed.

- Ideal Sleep Environment: Make sure your bedroom is cool, quiet, and dark.

- Limit Alcohol and Caffeine: Steer clear of alcohol and caffeine, especially after dark.

- Physical Activity: Exercise regularly can enhance sleep; however, avoid doing intense exercise right before bed.

- Nutrition and Diet: Pay attention to what you eat right before bed. Spicy or heavy meals can cause sleep disturbances.

- Control Stress: Stress reduction techniques can greatly improve the quality of your sleep.

- Limit Naps: Short naps during the day might be rejuvenating, but prolonged naps can disrupt your sleep at night.

- Speak with a Healthcare Professional: See a healthcare professional for advice and possible treatments if you constantly struggle with sleep issues.

In conclusion, good sleep hygiene and stress management are essential for general health, including breast health. By doing these things, you can lower your chance of developing breast cancer and help the body's innate capacity to stay healthy and fend against illness.

Through the integration of stress management strategies and the enhancement of sleep hygiene, people can enable themselves to actively participate in their breast health and general well-being.

Chapter 4: Breast Cancer Risk Factors And Prevention

A . Genetic and Environmental Risk Factors for Breast Cancer

Breast Cancer Risk Factors: Genetic and Environmental

Environmental and genetic variables work together to influence the risk of breast cancer. It is imperative to comprehend these risk factors to make well-informed decisions regarding early identification, screening, and prevention.

The following summarizes the environmental and genetic risk factors for breast cancer:

Risk Factors for Genetics

1. Family History: A family history of breast cancer is a substantial genetic risk factor, particularly if a first-degree relative (mother, sister, or daughter) had the disease. Particular gene mutations, such as those in BRCA1 and BRCA2, greatly raise the risk.

2. Mutations in the BRCA1 or BRCA2 genes: These mutations greatly increase the risk of breast cancer if inherited. These mutations are detectable by genetic testing.

3. Additional Genetic Mutations: Variations in genes including TP53, ATM, CHEK2, and PALB2 can potentially raise the chance of developing breast cancer.

4. Family Cancer Syndromes: There is an increased risk of breast cancer in those with certain rare genetic syndromes, such as Cowden syndrome and Li-Fraumeni syndrome.

5. Age and Gender: Two non-modifiable risk factors for breast cancer include becoming older and being feminine.

Environmental Risk Factors

1. Long-term usage of mixed estrogen and progesterone HRT has been associated with a higher risk of breast cancer. Talking about the advantages and disadvantages of a medical professional is crucial.

2. Reproductive and Hormonal Factors: Early menstruation, late menopause, not having children or having children later in life, and using birth control pills can all have an impact on the risk of breast cancer.

3. Radiation Exposure: Receiving radiation therapy to the chest in the past, especially in childhood or adolescence, may raise your risk.

4. Alcohol Consumption: Drinking too much alcohol has been linked to a higher risk of breast cancer.

5. Lifestyle Factors: Adopting unhealthy habits like smoking, eating poorly, not exercising, and being obese can raise your chance of developing breast cancer.

6. Diet: A diet low in fruits and vegetables and high in processed foods and saturated fats may put a person at risk.

7. Breast Density: Because dense breast tissue can make it more difficult to see cancers on mammograms, women who have it may be at increased risk.

8. Environmental Toxins: Although more research is required in this area, exposure to endocrine-disrupting chemicals and environmental pollutants may increase the risk of breast cancer.

9. Menstrual and Reproductive History: Early onset of menstruation and late menopause can lead to increased estrogen exposure and an increased risk of breast cancer.

10. Physical Inactivity: There is a larger risk when there is a lack of consistent physical activity.

It's crucial to remember that while these risk factors contribute to the development of breast cancer, possessing one or more of them does not ensure that a person will get the disease. Furthermore, a large number of women who have breast cancer do not have any known risk factors. Breast health is mostly dependent on lifestyle decisions, early identification, and routine screening. Speak with a healthcare professional for advice on early detection and prevention of breast cancer as well as a specific risk assessment.

B. Hormone Replacement Therapy (HRT)

To replace the hormones that the body may no longer manufacture in sufficient amounts, especially during and after menopause, hormone replacement therapy (HRT) entails taking drugs that include hormones, such as progesterone and estrogen. Although hormone replacement therapy (HRT) has many advantages, there are hazards and things to keep in mind. This is a synopsis:

Advantages:

1. Relief from Menopausal Symptoms: Hormone replacement therapy (HRT) is a very successful treatment for hot flashes, vaginal dryness, night sweats, and mood swings.

2. Bone Health: HRT, especially in postmenopausal women, can help preserve bone density and lower the risk of osteoporosis and fractures.

3. Cardiovascular Health: By lowering the risk of heart disease and raising cholesterol levels, hormone replacement therapy (HRT) may occasionally be beneficial to heart health. Individual differences may exist, nevertheless, in this effect.

4. Vaginal Health: By reducing vaginal atrophy, HRT can improve the comfort of sexual activity.

Disadvantages:

1. Risk of Breast Cancer: One of the biggest issues with HRT is the potential for increased breast cancer risk, especially after long-term use. The kind of HRT, how long it lasts, and individual risk factors are some of

the variables that affect how much danger there is.

2. Blood Clots: Taking HRT may increase the chance of blood clots forming in veins, which may result in pulmonary embolism or deep vein thrombosis (DVT).

3. Stroke: Some research indicates that HRT may marginally raise the risk of stroke, particularly in postmenopausal women.

4. Heart Disease: While some women may benefit from hormone replacement therapy (HRT), not all women are candidates. Individual characteristics and the kind of HRT used can have an impact on the risk of heart disease.

5. Endometrial cancer: There may be a higher risk of endometrial cancer in women who take estrogen without progesterone. Progesterone and estrogen together can lower this risk.

6. Gallbladder Disease: The chance of gallbladder disease may increase with HRT.

7. Memory and Cognitive Health: Research on how HRT affects cognitive performance and the risk of dementia is ongoing, although results have been inconsistent.

8. The selection of hormone type (such as synthetic or bioidentical) and delivery mechanism (such as tablets, patches, creams, or gels) might have

an impact on the advantages and disadvantages of hormone replacement therapy.

Observations and Recommendations:

1 . Tailored Approach: Each person should make their own decisions on HRT. To determine your symptoms, medical history, and risk factors, speak with a healthcare professional.

2. Minimum Adequate Dose: In cases when hormone replacement therapy (HRT) is considered suitable, medical professionals frequently advise utilizing the lowest effective dosage for the shortest amount of time required to relieve menopausal symptoms.

3. Frequent Health Check-ups: To monitor their health and address any changes or concerns, women on hormone replacement therapy should schedule routine follow-up consultations with their healthcare physician.

4. Options: Dietary adjustments, lifestyle adjustments, and non-hormonal therapies can help control menopausal symptoms and may be more suited for some people.

5. Shared Decision-Making: Taking into account your particular health profile and preferences, you and your healthcare provider should jointly decide whether to begin or continue HRT.

In conclusion, hormone replacement therapy may be a useful choice for treating some medical issues and easing menopausal symptoms. But using HRT carries hazards, so it's important to consider your personal preferences and circumstances before deciding to use it. Maintaining regular contact with a healthcare professional is crucial for tracking the advantages and possible hazards of hormone replacement therapy.

C. Techniques for Risk Reduction

Techniques for Lowering the Risk of Breast Cancer

It takes a combination of healthy lifestyle decisions, routine screenings, and knowledge of personal risk factors to lower the chance of breast cancer. The following are methods for lowering the risk of breast cancer:

1. Frequent Examination and Prompt Identification:

- Mammograms: If you have risk factors, start screening for breast cancer at age 40 or earlier, and adhere to prescribed mammography recommendations.

- Clinical Breast Exams: Include clinical breast exams in your routine physicals.

2. Self-Examinations at Breast:

- Conduct self-breast inspections every month to familiarize yourself with your breast tissue. Notify your healthcare physician right away if anything changes.

3. Recognize Your Risks:

- Recognize the risk variables that affect you, such as genetics, family history, and hormones.

4. Nutritious Food and Nutrition:

- Opt for a diet that is well-balanced and abundant in whole grains, fruits, vegetables, lean meats, and healthy fats.

- Restrict or stay away from processed foods, foods heavy in fat and sugar, and excessive alcohol use.

5. Engaging in Exercise:

- Get regular exercise, trying to get in at least 150 minutes a week of moderate-intensity or 75 minutes a week of vigorous-intensity exercise.

6. Maintaining Weight:

- Balance your calorie consumption and physical activity to maintain a healthy body weight.

- Being overweight is a known risk factor for breast cancer, particularly after menopause.

7. Drinking in Moderation:

If you drink, restrict how much you drink or drink in moderation since drinking too much alcohol raises your risk of developing breast cancer.

8. Nursing a baby:

- Breastfeeding is related to a lower incidence of breast cancer, therefore try to do it if you can for your kids.

9. Treatment with Hormone Replacement (HRT):

-To control symptoms, use the lowest effective dose for the shortest amount of time after speaking with your healthcare professional about the benefits and dangers of hormone replacement therapy.

10. Avoid Toxins in the Environment:

- Take precautions to avoid exposure to chemicals that disrupt hormones and environmental contaminants. Reduce your exposure to potentially dangerous substances.

11. Stress Reduction:

- Use stress-reduction strategies to lessen the effects of ongoing stress, such as deep breathing, exercise, or meditation.

12. Restful Sleep:

-Make getting a good night's sleep a priority by adhering to a regular sleep schedule, setting up a cozy sleeping space, and using appropriate sleep hygiene.

13. Frequent Medical Examinations:

- See your doctor for routine check-ups so that they can evaluate your general health and talk to you about breast health.

14. Genetic Testing and Counseling:

- You should think about genetic counseling and testing for inherited gene mutations like BRCA1 and BRCA2 if you have a strong family history of breast cancer or other risk factors.

15. Assistance and Instruction:

- Look for information and assistance from breast cancer organizations and reliable sources.

- Keep up with the most recent findings and advice regarding breast health.

16. Assessment of Breast Density:

- Talk to your healthcare provider about additional screening alternatives such as breast ultrasonography or 3D mammography if you have dense breast tissue.

17. Hormonal Birth Control:

-If you are worried about the link between breast cancer risk and hormonal contraception, consider using non-hormonal birth control options.

Keep in mind that while implementing these tactics will lower your chance of developing breast cancer, no strategy can ensure total prevention. Reducing the risk of breast cancer is a proactive and all-encompassing endeavor that combines lifestyle decisions, routine screenings, and well-informed decision-making in collaboration with healthcare professionals.

Chapter 5: Support and Treatment Options

A. Types of Breast cancer

Breast cancer comes in a variety of forms, each with unique traits.

The following are the most typical forms of breast cancer:

1. Ductal Carcinoma In Situ (DCIS): This non-invasive malignancy is identified by abnormal cells in the breast duct lining. Being the most common type of breast cancer, it is usually quite curable.

2. Invasive Ductal Carcinoma (IDC): The most prevalent kind of breast

cancer is IDC. It starts in the milk ducts and spreads to the breast's surrounding tissues. It has the potential to spread to other bodily parts.

3. Lobular Carcinoma Invasive (ILC): ILC can expand to other areas of the breast and the body, beginning in the lobules, the glands that produce milk.

4. Triple-Negative Breast Cancer: HER2/neu receptors, progesterone, and estrogen are absent in this subtype of breast cancer. It may have few alternatives for treatment and tends to be more aggressive.

5. HER2-Positive Breast Cancer: This type of breast cancer is usually more aggressive than overexpressing the

HER2/neu gene. Treatments for this kind of condition include targeted medications like Herceptin.

6. Inflammatory Breast Cancer: This is an uncommon and highly aggressive type of disease. It tends to spread swiftly and frequently manifests as breast swelling and redness, similar to inflammation.

7. Male Breast Cancer: Although it affects women far more frequently, men can also get breast cancer; typically, it manifests as IDC or ILC.

8. Metastatic Breast Cancer: This is metastatic breast cancer that has spread to other bodily organs including the liver, lungs, or bones. It is not a separate type of breast cancer.

It is significant to remember that hormone receptor status (progesterone and estrogen receptors) and HER2 status (which affects therapy choices) are additional characteristics that can be used to further categorize breast cancer. Selecting the best course of treatment depends heavily on the unique forms and traits of breast cancer.

To determine the subtype of breast cancer and develop a successful treatment strategy, you or someone you know must collaborate closely with a medical team.

B. Modalities of treatment

Breast Cancer Treatment Options

The kind, stage, and other unique characteristics of breast cancer all influence the course of treatment. For the best results, a variety of therapeutic techniques are frequently utilized in combination. The following are the main methods of treating breast cancer:

1.   Surgery: -   Lumpectomy (Breast-Conserving Surgery): This procedure preserves the majority of the breast while removing the tumor and a narrow margin of surrounding tissue.

- Mastectomy: involves removing the entire breast, occasionally along with the lymph nodes that surround it.

- Sentinel Lymph Node Biopsy: Identifies whether cancer has progressed to lymph nodes in the vicinity.

- Axillary Lymph Node Dissection: This procedure involves removing several lymph nodes from the armpit for additional testing.

- Reconstructive Surgery: To restore the look of the breast after mastectomy.

2. Radiation therapy: - Targets and destroys cancer cells or lowers the chance of recurrence using high-energy X-rays.

3. Chemotherapy: Often used for more aggressive or advanced breast tumors, chemotherapy uses medications to either kill or halt the growth of cancer cells.

4. Hormone therapy: - Reduces or blocks the amounts of progesterone and estrogen, which are the main hormones driving hormone receptor-positive breast tumors.

- Frequently applied to breast tumors that are ER-positive, or estrogen receptor-positive. Tamoxifen, aromatase inhibitors (such as letrozole and anastrozole), and other medications are among them.

5. Targeted Therapy: - Targets particular chemicals or pathways that contribute to the development of cancer.

- Treatments for HER2-positive breast tumors include Herceptin, Pertuzumab, and T-DM1. These are HER2-targeted treatments.

-Combining hormone therapy with other targeted medicines such as CDK4/6 inhibitors (e.g., Palbociclib, Ribociclib) is common practice.

6. Immunotherapy: A more recent strategy that strengthens the body's defenses against cancer by stimulating the immune system; frequently used in clinical studies.

7. Neoadjuvant Therapy: - A treatment to reduce tumor size is administered before surgery.

8. Adjuvant Therapy: Post-surgery, treatment is administered to lower the chance of cancer recurrence.

- Incorporates hormone therapy, targeted therapy, chemotherapy, and radiation therapy.

9. Supportive Care: - Provides pain relief, anti-nausea drugs, and emotional support to address symptoms and side effects of treatment.

10. Palliative Care: - aims to enhance the quality of life for patients suffering

from metastatic or advanced breast cancer.

- Offers emotional support and symptom management.

The choice of treatment modalities is based on several variables, including the cancer's stage, grade, molecular characteristics, and the patient's general health and preferences. The patient, oncologists, surgeons, and other medical professionals frequently work together to create treatment programs.

The objective is to treat breast cancer as effectively and individually as possible while reducing side effects and maintaining quality of life.

C. Social and emotional assistance

Social and emotional support are essential for people coping with breast cancer. It can be very difficult to deal with the psychological, emotional, and physical effects of a breast cancer diagnosis and treatment. Here are some strategies to look for and offer social and emotional support:

Seeking Assistance:

1. Family and Friends: Seek out emotional support from those close to you. During this trying time, they can offer solace, support, and friendship.

2. Support Groups: Attend life or virtually-based support groups for

women with breast cancer. These groups provide a secure environment for others who are traveling similar paths to exchange stories, worries, and advice.

3. Mental Health Professionals: To treat the emotional effects of breast cancer, think about therapy or counseling. You can handle stress, depression, and anxiety with the aid of a mental health expert.

4. Online Communities: Engage in breast cancer-related chat rooms, social media groups, and online forums. These platforms give you access to a large group of people who are sympathetic to your situation.

5. Patient Navigators: Social workers or patient navigators are available at many healthcare facilities. They can offer emotional support, information, and connections to services.

6. Religious or Spiritual Communities: Seeking assistance from your religious community can be consoling and inspiring for individuals who identify as religious or spiritual.

Providing Assistance:

1. Be a Good Listener: Pay attention to the person receiving support if they have breast cancer. Give them space to communicate their emotions and worries without passing judgment.

2.   Empathy   and   Understanding: Exhibit understanding and empathy. Recognize their emotional journey and provide comfort.

3. Accompany to Appointments: Make an offer to go to your loved one's doctor's appointments, examinations, and therapies. The presence of a helpful person might lessen anxiety.

4. Help with Daily duties: To lessen the load, provide practical assistance with daily duties like cooking, cleaning, food shopping, or childcare.

5. Honor Their Choices: Honor their decisions about care, assistance, and lifestyle modifications. Provide advice and information, but respect their final choices.

6. Refrain from Giving unwanted Advice: Refrain from telling unfavorable tales or offering unwanted medical advice. Make an effort to create a welcoming and encouraging atmosphere.

7. Research Assistance: Provide support in looking up resources and treatment possibilities. Having an informed advocate can be very beneficial.

8. Encouragement: As a token of your concern and support, send encouraging letters, cards, or modest presents.

Keep in mind that social and emotional assistance are reciprocal. Open communication is necessary for the person with breast cancer and their support system to voice their needs and provide assistance. Establishing a robust support network can enhance the psychological welfare and general experience of individuals coping with breast cancer, rendering the ordeal more tolerable and less lonely.

Chapter 6: Real Stories and Testimonials

A. Individual narratives from breast cancer survivors

Individuals facing comparable circumstances might find inspiration, support, and vital insights from the personal accounts and tales of breast cancer survivors. The following well-known breast cancer survivors have opened up about their experiences:

1. Sheryl Crow: In 2006, the Grammy-winning vocalist and composer received a breast cancer diagnosis. She has fought for early

detection and increased public awareness of breast cancer.

2. Robin Roberts: In 2007, the ABC co-anchor of "Good Morning America" received a breast cancer diagnosis. She has been transparent about her experience and the value of routine tests.

3. Kylie Minogue: In 2005, the well-known Australian pop artist received a breast cancer diagnosis. She has made use of her platform to spread awareness of the illness.

4. Christina Applegate: In 2008, the comedian and actress received a breast cancer diagnosis. She has been a proponent of early detection and genetic testing.

5. Hoda Kotb: In 2007, the co-host of "Today Show" received a breast cancer diagnosis. She has urged people to get mammograms by sharing her personal experiences.

6. Giuliana Rancic: In 2011, the TV host and celebrity received a breast cancer diagnosis. She has been transparent about everything about her journey, even her choice to have a double mastectomy.

7. Rita Wilson: In 2015, the singer and actress received a breast cancer diagnosis. She has discussed the value of an early diagnosis and her personal experience.

8. Joan Lunden: In 2014, the former co-host of "Good Morning America"

received a breast cancer diagnosis. Through her blog, she has documented her journey and served as an advocate for breast cancer awareness.

Through their platforms, these survivors have encouraged early detection, increased public awareness of breast cancer, and offered encouragement and support to others. Their experiences serve as a reminder that while anybody can be affected by breast cancer, it is possible to overcome this difficult illness with early identification, appropriate treatment, and a strong support network.

B. Surmounting obstacles and discovering hope

Finding hope after receiving a breast cancer diagnosis is a path that calls for fortitude, resiliency, and support. The following techniques can assist those dealing with breast cancer in overcoming obstacles and finding hope:

1. Remain Informed: Information gives you power. Recognize your condition, available treatments, and any possible adverse effects. Make inquiries and look for information from trustworthy sources.

2. Create a Support System: Call on loved ones, close friends, support organizations, and medical professionals. Talking to someone about your worries and feelings might

help you feel better and be more positive.

3. Self-Care: Make self-care a priority to maintain your mental and physical health. This entails leading a healthy lifestyle, obtaining adequate sleep, and controlling your stress.

4. Establish Realistic Goals: Divide your journey into doable segments. Establish attainable objectives, no matter how big or tiny, to keep yourself feeling like you're making progress.

5. Emotional Expression: Use art, writing, or therapy sessions to communicate your feelings. This can lessen your anxiety and assist you in processing your emotions.

6. Mindfulness and Meditation: These techniques can lower stress and encourage inner peace and mental clarity.

7. Appreciate Little Victories: Acknowledge and rejoice in every accomplishment, regardless of how modest. Every advance is a triumph.

8. Find Inspiration: Read about the struggles and triumphs of breast cancer survivors. Their stories can reassure and encourage you.

9. Take Part in Positive Activities: Find interests and pastimes that make you happy and give your life a feeling of normalcy.

10.   Volunteer   or   Give   Back: Occasionally, giving to others can give one a feeling of direction and hope. Think   about   helping   out   or contributing to a good cause.

11.   Maintain Your Connection to Nature: Spending time outdoors, whether on walks or treks, may be calming and restorative.

12. Speak up for Yourself: Take an active role in your care and treatment. To make well-informed decisions, discuss your concerns, ask questions, and   work   together   with   your healthcare team.

13. Visualization and Affirmations: To cultivate a hopeful outlook, employ

visualization exercises and encouraging statements.

14. Make Future Plans: Continue to work toward your long-term objectives and dreams. Anticipating future events can inspire drive and hope.

15. Adopt Flexibility: Accept that there can be ups and downs on your path. It's acceptable to modify your expectations and goals as necessary.

16. Take into Account Professional Support: Don't be afraid to get professional assistance if you're having trouble managing your fear and anxiety. Counselors and therapists can offer techniques for controlling these feelings.

17. Make Connections with Other Survivors: Talk about Your Experiences and Take Advice from Those Who Have Beat Breast Cancer. They can provide emotional support as well as original insights.

Recall that pursuing hope is a continuous and individual activity. There will be times when you feel scared and uncertain, but you can overcome obstacles and welcome hope for the future if you have patience, perseverance, and a strong support system. Survivors of breast cancer frequently experience a greater sense of strength and gratitude for life.

Chapter 7: Additional Information Sources

A. Connections to reputable sites and businesses

The following reputable websites and groups offer helpful resources, support, and information on breast cancer:

1. American Cancer Society (ACS) - www.cancer.org is their website. The American Cancer Society (ACS) offers thorough information on breast cancer, including risk factors, prophylaxis, available treatments, and available support systems.

2.   Breastcancer.org: [www.breastcancer.org] is the website address. Breastcancer.org provides a plethora of information on breast cancer, including forums, a hotline, and current medical articles.

3. Komen for the Cure, Susan, the [www.komen.org]   website https://www.komen.org, The goals of this group include advocacy, education, and research on breast cancer. They provide support services and information on breast health.

4. The National Breast Cancer Foundation, Inc. (NBCF): https://www.nationalbreastcancer is the website address for individuals impacted by breast cancer, NBCF

offers information, tools, and support services for early detection.

5. The network for metastatic breast cancer (MBCN) http://www.mbcn.org/ The mission of MBCN is to help and educate people whose breast cancer has spread to other areas.

6. LBBC, or Living Beyond Breast Cancer: https://www.lbbc.org For individuals impacted by breast cancer, LBBC provides a network, support services, and instructional materials.

7. Breast Cancer Now (UK): [breast cancer now. org] is the website of a UK-based group that offers information on activism, support, and research related to breast cancer.

8. Young Survival Coalition (YSC): https://www.youngsurvival.org/ is the organization's website with an emphasis on the particular difficulties faced by young women receiving a breast cancer diagnosis, YSC provides resources and support from the community.

9. The National Cancer Institute's website, cancer.gov: [www.cancer.gov] On its website, the NCI offers comprehensive details about clinical trials, research, treatment choices, and breast cancer in general.

10. UK-Based Breast Cancer Care: [www.breastcancercare.org.uk] is the website UK-based group that provides breast cancer patients with

community, support services, and information.

Please be aware that although these groups and websites provide helpful information and assistance, you should always speak with medical professionals for specific recommendations and treatment alternatives.

Conclusion

A . Recap of key takeaways

The following is the summary of the main lessons learned about breast health, breast cancer, and support:

Breast Wellness:

1. Frequent self-examinations of the breast are crucial for early detection.

2. Mammograms and annual clinical breast exams are essential for screening.

3. Sustaining a nutritious diet and regular exercise promotes breast health.

4. Getting enough sleep and managing stress are essential to general well-being.

Maternal Cancer:

5. There are other kinds of breast cancer, such as triple-negative, HER2-positive, IDC, and ILC.

6. Environmental and genetic variables can affect the risk of breast cancer.

7. Surgery, radiation, chemotherapy, hormone therapy, targeted therapy,

and immunotherapy are some of the available treatment options.

8. Having social and emotional support is crucial when coping with breast cancer.

Overcoming Obstacles and Discovering Hope:

9. It's critical to maintain knowledge and create a support system.

10. It's critical to engage in self-care and to seek expert assistance when necessary.

11. Little triumphs and constructive endeavors give rise to hope.

12. You can lower your stress levels by practicing mindfulness, meditation, and creative expression.

13. It is empowering to make plans and set reasonable goals.

14. Making connections with other survivors might offer insightful perspectives and psychological assistance.

Reliable sources:

15. A wealth of information and support is available from organizations like Susan G. Komen, Breastcancer.org, the American Cancer Society, and others.

16. Comprehensive information is available through government health resources like the National Cancer Institute.

17. Worldwide groups such as Breast Cancer Now (UK) provide research information and assistance.

Keep in mind that controlling breast health and treating breast cancer require information, early detection, and support. Speak with medical specialists for individualized advice and available treatments.

B. Proactive promotion of breast health

Yes, let me offer some motivation for proactive breast health:

1. Know Your Body: Preventive breast health begins with an awareness of your breasts and how they normally feel and appear. Examine your breasts regularly to look for any changes.

2. Early Detection Prevents Death: Clinical breast exams and mammograms are crucial for early detection. These screenings can detect breast cancer in its most curable phases, so don't put them off.

3. Keep Up a Healthy Lifestyle: Eating a balanced diet and doing regular exercise improve general health and may lower the chance of breast cancer.

4. You're Not Alone: Keep in mind that there are organizations, support groups, and medical specialists available to assist you at every stage if you ever have worries about your breast health.

5. Accept Empowerment: Taking charge of your breast health gives you power. Your level of awareness and what you do can have a big impact on your well-being.

6. Self-Care Matters: Give self-care top priority. Taking care of yourself, getting enough sleep, and doing constructive things are essential for resilience and general health.

7. Information Is Power: Learn as much as you can about breast health

and breast cancer. Knowing is essential for making wise selections.

8. Appreciate Little Wins: Every action you do to maintain proactive breast health is a win. Rejoice in your accomplishments and keep going.

9. Support is Available: Those embarking on a breast health journey can find a multitude of support and encouragement from friends, family, and committed organizations.

You are investing in your future and well-being when you take a proactive approach to breast health. You're taking action to safeguard your health by being proactive because it matters.